A Quick Guide to Children's Oral Health

ALYSSA WALKER GLOSSON, RDH

Text & Illustrations by Alyssa Walker Glosson

Copyright © 2015 Alyssa Walker Glosson

ISBN-13: 978-1511782715
ISBN-10: 1511782714

INTRODUCTION

Cavities Don't Have to Happen! Clean teeth don't get cavities. Having seen many young patients with unnecessary decay, who have not been practicing good dental habits, I have been inspired to provide some very quick and basic information on oral care. Proper care at home and regular visits to your dentist and dental hygienist can result in a lasting, healthy smile. This is dedicated to anyone who is concerned with helping a child learn the habits necessary to achieve a lifetime of good oral hygiene.

-Alyssa Walker Glosson, RDH

CONTENTS

I   Why Bother to Care for Baby Teeth   1

First Tooth   2

First Dental Visit   2

Early Childhood Caries and Feeding   3

Pacifier and Thumb Sucking   4

Fluoride   4

Bottled Water and Fluoride   5

Chewing Gum   6

Medications   6

Overall Health   6

Dental Health on a Budget   7

II   Daily Bacterial Plaque Removal   8

Caring for Baby's Gums   8

Brushing and Flossing   8

Brushing & Flossing Technique   10

To Rinse or Not to Rinse   11

Sealants   11

Conclusion   12

Sources   15

A Quick Guide to Children's Oral Health

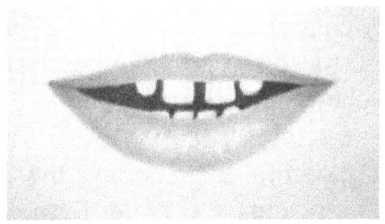

Goal: A child free of caries (cavities) with optimum
gingival (gum) health.

**Why bother to care for primary (baby) teeth, since they
are going to fall out?**

It seems natural to question why it is important to care for
the "baby" teeth, since they will fall out anyway. Children
need good oral health. Decay in baby, or primary, teeth
often leads to the start of decay in the permanent teeth as
they eventually start to come in. Also, if oral health issues
become severe at any age, they can have a negative effect
on the overall health of the individual. In addition to these,
there are other reasons to begin good habits at an early age.
The primary teeth could be looked at as a set of "practice"
teeth. If a child begins the habit of neglecting his teeth at a
young age, it is much less likely that he will build the
habits needed to care for his permanent teeth- at least not
before he has learned the lesson the hard way with some
dental caries (cavities) in the permanent set. However,
good dental routines and habits practiced daily can lead to a
lifelong healthy smile.

Primary teeth also serve as the foundation for healthy gums and the proper positioning of permanent teeth. They are natural space maintainers, holding the space open until the permanent teeth are ready to take their place. When a baby tooth is lost too early, the permanent teeth can drift into the empty space making it difficult for other adult teeth to find room when they come in. This can make teeth crowded or crooked, leading to costly orthodontics. Baby teeth also help your child chew and speak clearly.

The practice of good oral hygiene lays the foundation of a healthy mouth and helps the child form habits of good dental care which can lead to a lifetime of good dental health.

First Tooth

The average age for the first primary (baby) tooth is 5 - 6 months; however, there can be variations for each individual.

First Dental Visit

The first visit should occur within six months after the first tooth erupts, but no later than the child's first birthday. Regular visits allow for oral assessment and aid in prevention of cavities. Furthermore, this helps the child learn to not fear seeing the dentist or hygienist. This is an important step in a lifetime of good oral health.

Early Childhood Caries and Feeding

Early childhood caries (ECC), also known as baby bottle cavities, baby bottle tooth decay, or bottle rot, is severe decay in the teeth of infants. It is a common infectious bacterial disease from Streptococcus Mutans (cariogenic bacteria). It is commonly caused by sweetened liquids and also by any saliva sharing activity such as, tasting food before feeding, sharing eating utensils, sucking on a pacifier to clean it, etc.... It is best to avoid routinely giving a bottle when putting the child to sleep, because the liquid collects around the teeth causing demineralization (weakening of the enamel), which can result in decay.

o   It is best to never start giving your child a bottle at bedtime.

o   If a bottle is used, avoid sweet juices or milk, use only water.

o   It is recommended that babies' and toddler's teeth and gums be cleaned after every meal starting from their teeth's first emergence.

o   It is best to discontinue bottle feeding altogether by at least the age of twelve months and begin using cups for drinking. The use of a cup not only helps develop coordination skills, but helps prevent misalignment as the teeth and mouth develop.

Pacifier and Thumb Sucking

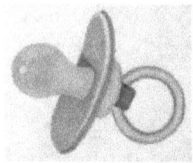 While sucking on a thumb or pacifier is a natural reflex, prolonged thumb sucking may cause problems with the proper growth and development of the mouth and the alignment of the teeth. It is thought by some that sucking on a pacifier doesn't do as much damage as the thumb would; however, the American Dental Association (ADA) has determined that it can affect the teeth in essentially the same way. You may talk to your child's dentist or hygienist about their thoughts on this issue. Most children stop between 2-4 years old. If it has not stopped before the age of four, it should be discouraged at that time.

o   Don't pressure the child; instead, encourage them to give it up by setting a positive tone.

o   Give plenty of praise when the child isn't sucking their thumb.

o   If your child continues to suck their thumb, talk to your dentist or pediatrician.

Fluoride

Fluoride should be in the infant's daily diet for proper mineralization of the bones and teeth. Exposure to fluoride during infancy helps prevent tooth decay. In most cases, you can safely use fluoridated tap water to prepare infant formula.

Even though fluoride helps to control and prevent tooth decay, too much fluoride from water or other fluoride sources, such as toothpastes in the early years when teeth are developing (from birth – age 8), can have negative effects. It can cause changes in the appearance of the tooth's surface, known as dental fluorosis, which is a mottling of the teeth, causing a white chalky appearance of the enamel. This gradually undergoes a brown discoloration.

There has been some debate about the impact of fluoride on general health concerns. There have been many studies on the safety of fluoride use. Studies have shown that when the exposure to fluoride is not greater than the standard set by the Environmental Protection Agency (EPA), there is no evidence that it is unsafe. Fluoride still remains the most effective way to prevent tooth decay, especially in individuals who have a high-risk for decay. Contact your child's dentist or pediatrician for fluoride recommendations that are best suited for your child. If fluoride use remains a concern, there are non-fluoride toothpastes available.

Bottled Water and Fluoride

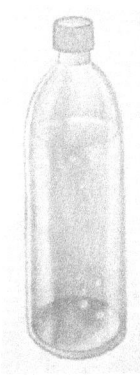

Many people only drink bottled water, but bottled water does not have the recommended levels of fluoride contained in most tap water. Many children may not receive the same anti-cavity benefits as those who consume tap water. Ask your child's dental professional about the fluoride levels in the water source in your area, and they can provide the best recommendation for oral health by taking into account the type and quantity of water your child drinks.

Chewing Gum

Once the child is old enough to chew gum, select a gum that reduces the harmful effects of sugar. Sugar free gums are a good choice to reduce the harmful, decay causing effects of sugar. An even better choice is a gum containing xylitol, which is a natural alternative for sugar. Xylitol actually helps prevent decay and provides oral therapeutic benefits by reducing the buildup of plaque and harmful acids in the child's mouth.

Medications

Many medications are made with a sugar or syrupy base to disguise the bad flavor. You can request or purchase sugar-free medicine if available, especially if it is a long-term medicine. When it does not interfere with the efficacy of the drug, rinse and brush the child's mouth with clean water immediately after the medication is given to counteract the negative result of sugars on the teeth.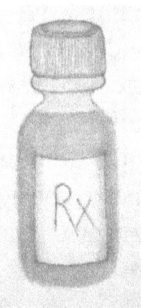

Overall Health

There is a connection between the health of a person's mouth, teeth, and gums and their overall health. Without proper oral hygiene, bacteria in the mouth can reach levels that may contribute or lead to other infections and diseases throughout the rest of the body. Taking care of oral health is an investment in one's overall physical wellbeing.

Also, by eating a healthy diet, drinking more water, and

limiting sugary foods, a person can not only improve their overall health but also increase their chances of maintaining good oral hygiene.

Dental Health on a Budget

Even if you have a very limited budget and regular dental visits are difficult for you to afford, maintaining good dental hygiene can save you money in the long run. Practicing good dental care at home will reduce the number of problems that will occur as the child grows up.

If finances are tight, look for opportunities in your community for reduced cost or free dental care for your child. Some dentists will work out a payment plan if you cannot initially afford the full price of treatment. If your local college or technical school has a dental program, dental hygiene program, or dental assisting program, they may offer free or low cost care for children (and adults), such as exams, dental cleanings, sealants, fillings, or extractions. There also may be a program sponsored by dentists in your area which offers free services for low income families on certain days of the year. Check with your local dentist, doctor, or health clinic for information on these and other services.

Daily Bacterial Plaque Removal

Caring for Baby's Gums

Until the first tooth erupts, gently use a soft, moistened washcloth or gauze to wipe the oral tissue and gingiva (gums) at least twice per day, especially after feeding and before bedtime.

As teeth are coming in, you can give your baby a clean cool teething ring to chew on when they are experiencing pain from teeth trying to make their way through their gums.

Brushing and Flossing

Children should brush a minimum of two times a day. A good habit is to brush in the morning and again before bed.

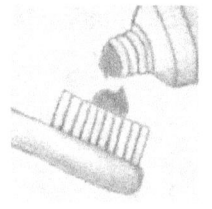 When the first tooth erupts, use a soft toothbrush designed for children. For children up to 3 years old, place a fluoride containing toothpaste (size of a grain of rice) on the toothbrush. For children 3-6 years of age use no more than a pea-sized amount of fluoride containing toothpaste on the toothbrush to brush twice per day. Brushing should last for two minutes; then, the child should spit out the toothpaste (don't let them swallow it). Replace the child's toothbrush every three to four months, or sooner if the bristles begin to fray.

There are many good toothbrushes, but electric toothbrushes with a two-minute timer are perfect for children. Electric toothbrushes can be fun for children to use, and may make them more likely to think of brushing as enjoyable. Also, digital or hour-glass style timers can be found in many colors or in fun character shapes, which can add additional excitement to daily brushing.

Just as with brushing, daily flossing for very young children will have to be done by the parent. As they mature and their motor skills develop, they can be taught to do it themselves. Waxed floss makes it easier to floss between teeth. Disposable flossers are great and 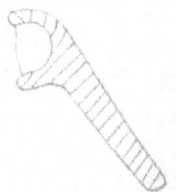 can make things go easier. If the child's teeth are hard to get floss between, there are other interdental cleaners, such as specially designed dental floss picks or water flossers for children, that can help clean between teeth (however, water flossers cannot fully replace floss for cleaning between teeth). It is not unusual for there to be a little bleeding near the gums when flossing is first begun, since the gums are not used to this. As flossing is done on a regular basis, instances of bleeding will decrease. If they do not, talk to your dental professional.

It is important that the child learn the proper way to brush and floss their teeth (the child's hygienist or dentist can demonstrate the proper technique). Children should usually be able to brush and floss themselves by the age of six or seven.

Brushing & Flossing Technique

When brushing, make small gentle circles as you work across all surfaces of the teeth. Brush the facial (outside), lingual (inside), and occlusal (top) surfaces. Finish by brushing the tongue, which also needs to be cleaned of the bacteria which causes tooth decay.

When flossing, gently move the floss back and forth as you work it down between the teeth. Guide the floss all the way down to the gum line. Work the floss up and down on the side of each tooth. Then, gently work it back up.

TIPS:
- An electric toothbrush takes away a lot of the uncertainty associated with manual brushing because it's moving continuously.

- The use of disclosing agents (chewable tablets, mouth rinses, or swabs which leave behind color to highlight remaining food or plaque) help the child to see the areas that he may be missing when brushing.

- It is best to monitor your child to make sure he is brushing and flossing correctly.

- The use of "fun" products like kids electric toothbrushes and disposable flossers help children learn to enjoy brushing and flossing their teeth and help them feel that they are in charge of their own oral health routines.

To Rinse or Not To Rinse after Brushing

Although this may come as a shock to some, not everyone agrees about whether or not one should rinse after brushing. There are valid arguments on both sides. On one hand, rinsing washes away all the bacteria just brushed off the teeth. However, on the other hand, rinsing also washes away some of the fluoride protecting benefits from the toothpaste.

I personally rinse the bacteria away after brushing my teeth, however, there could be additional benefits to allowing the fluoride to remain longer. If the dentist has informed you of some incipient caries (early stages of decay) on the child's teeth, then perhaps not rinsing away the fluoride could help reverse those small cavities. However, there is another option to increase the benefits of fluoride and still rinse away the bacteria.

After rinsing the bacteria away, children over the age of six could then rinse with a fluoride mouth rinse or use a fluoride supplement (fluoride mouth rinse is not recommended for children under six). It is important that the child not swallow the rinse, as swallowing too much fluoride can result in dental fluorosis. The child should then wait thirty minutes after using fluoride before eating or drinking to get the maximum benefit. Talk to your dental professional about selecting a fluoride rinse for your child.

Sealants

Pit and fissure sealants help protect the grooves and pits in the chewing surfaces of permanent posterior (back) teeth. Applications should be made as soon as possible. When it is delayed, cavities may start, preventing the surface from being a candidate for sealants. Because occlusal (top) surfaces are more vulnerable to decay than the facial and lingual (outside and inside) surfaces, extra protection is needed. The incidence of new pit and fissure cavities can be significantly lowered by the application of adhesive sealants.

In some cases, sealants may be appropriate for baby teeth. Since baby teeth are important for holding the correct placing for permanent teeth, it is important to care for these teeth and keep them healthy so they do not fall out too early.

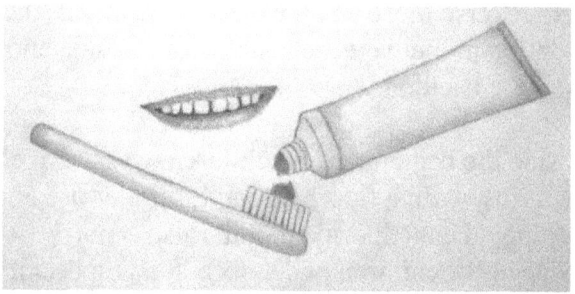

Conclusion:

Following these quick guidelines can help your child remain cavity free and maintain a nice healthy smile, and it may also save you money on your child's future dental visits. Practicing these steps regularly will also build habits for a lifetime of good oral health.

Happy Brushing!

SOURCES

Adair S, Bowen W, Burt B, Kumar J, Levy S, Pendrys D, Rozier RG, Selwitz RH, Stamm J, Stookey G. Recommendations for Using Fluoride to Prevent and Control Dental Caries in the United States. Mortality and Morbidity Report, http://www.cdc.gov/mmwr/preview/mmwrhtml/rr5014a1.htm, August 17, 2001.

Babies and Kids. Mouth Healthy, American Dental Association, http://www.mouth healthy.org/en/babies-and-kids/, 2014.

Baby Teeth. Mouth Healthy. American Dental Association, http://www.mouthhealthy.org/en/az-topics/b/baby-teeth, 2014.

Basic Information About Fluoride in Drinking Water. United States Environmental Protection Agency, http://water.epa.gov/drink/contaminants/basicinformation/fluoride.cfm, July 23, 2013.

Biesbrock AR, Faller RV, Bartizek RD, Court LK, McClanahan SF. Reversal of incipient and radiographic caries through the use of sodium and stannous fluoride dentifrices in a clinical trial. National Center for Biotechnology Information, U.S. National Library of Medicine, http://www.ncbi.nlm.nih.gov/pubmed/9835826, 1998.

Bradley M, Kinirons MJ. Provision of Sugar Free Medicines for Young Children: The Views of a Sample of Parents in North Ireland. National Center for Biotechnology Information, U.S. National Library of Medicine, http://www.ncbi.nlm.nih.gov/pubmed/9863440, 1998.

Broadbent J, Thompson WM, Ramrakha S, Moffit T, Zeng J, Page LA, Poulton R. Community Water Fluoridation and Intelligence: Prospective Study in New Zealand. American Journal of Public Health, http://ajph.aphapublications.org/doi/abs/10.2105/AJPH.201 3.301857, December 20, 2013.

Brushing & Flossing.http://www.pediatricdentistry ct.com/PatientInformation/BrushingFlossing/tabid/81/ Default.aspx, 2009.

Cavities/Tooth Decay: Prevention. Mayo Foundation for Medical Education and Research, http://www.mayo clinic.org/diseases-conditions/cavities/basics/prevention/ con-20030076, May 30, 2014.

Clark S. Wonders of Xylitol. RDH, http://www.rdh mag.com/articles/print/volume-31/issue4/features/wonders-of-xylitol.html, 2015.

Council on Clinical Affairs. Guideline on Caries Risk Assessment and Management for Infants, Children, and Adolescents. American Academy of Pediatric Dentistry, http://www.aapd.org/media/Policies_Guidelines/G_CariesR iskAssessment.pdf, 2002, revised 2014: 127 – 134.

DaSilva JD. Oxford American Handbook of Clinical Dentistry. Oxford University Press, 2008: 28-31.

Dental Exam for Children. Mayo Foundation for Medical Education and Research, http://www.mayo clinic.org/tests-procedures/dental-exam-forchildren/basics/why-its-done/prc-20013782, February 18, 2012.

Driscoll WS, Swango PA, Horowitz AM, Kingman A. Carries-Preventative Effects of Daily and Weekly Fluoride Mouthrinsing in an Optimally Fluoridated Community: Findings After Eighteen Months. Pediatric Dentistry Vol. 3 No. 4, http://www.aapd.org/assets/1/25/ Driscoll-03-04.pdf, 1981: 316 – 320.

Drop those Pacifiers! American Dental Association, http://www.ada.org/en/press-room/news-releases/2013-archive/may/drop-those-pacifiers, May 6, 2013.

Eakle WS. Thumb Sucking. Health Encyclopedia, Baylor Health Care System, http://healthsource.baylor health.com/Library/Encyclopedia/90,P01875, March 31, 2013.

Fast Facts. American Academy of Pediatric Dentistry, http://www.aapd.org/assets/1/7/FastFacts.pdf, 2014.

Fawell J, Bailey K, Chilton J, Dahi E, Fewtrell L, Magara Y. Fluoride in Drinking Water. World Health Organization, http://www.who.int/water_sanitation_health/publications/ fluoride_drinking_water_full.pdf., 2006.

Fluoride and Fluoridation. American Dental Association, http://www.ada.org/en/publicprograms/ advocating-for-the-public/fluoride-and-fluoridation, 2014.

Fluoride Facts. American Dental Hygienists' Association, http://www.adha.org/sites/default/files/ 7253_Fluoride_Facts.pdf, 2015.

Fluoridation Safety. Division of Oral Health, National Center for Chronic Disease Prevention and Health Promotion, http://www.cdc.gov/fluoridation/safety/ index.htm, July 10, 2013.

Fluoride Supplements. American Dental Association, http://wwhw.ada.org/en/member-center/oral-healthtopics/ fluoride-supplements, 2010.

Fluorosis. Mouth Healthy, http://www.mouth healthy.org/en/az-topics/f/fluorosis, 2014.

For the Dental Patient: Facts About Bottled Water. Journal of the America Dental Association, Vol. 134, http://www.ada.org/~/media/ADA/Member%20Center/ FIles/patient_30.ashx, August 2003: 1287.

For the Dental Patient: Taking Care of Your Child's Smile. Journal of the America Dental Association, Vol. 145(5), http://www.ada.org/~/media/ADA/Publications/ Files/ForthePatient-0514.ashx, May 2014: 504.

For the Dental Patient: Thumb Sucking and Pacifier Use. Journal of the America Dental Association, Vol. 138, http://www.ada.org/~/media/ADA/Publications/Files/patien t_77.ashx, August 2007.

Gelberg KH, Fitzgerald EF, Hwang SA, Dubrow R. Fluoride Exposure and Childhood Osteosarcoma: A Case-Control Study. American Journal of Public Health, Vol. 85, No. 12, http://ajph.aphapublications.org/doi/abs/10.2 105/AJPH.85.12.1678, December 1995: 1678 - 1683.

Glazer H. Treating White Spots: New Caries Infiltration Technique. Dentistry Today, http://www. dentistrytoday.com/restorative/minimally-invasive-dentistry/1492, 2015.

Hoecker JL. Infant and Toddler Health: Is It Safe to Mix Fluoridated Tap Water with Infant Formula? I've Heard that Too Much Fluoride Can Harm a Baby's Teeth. Mayo Foundation for Medical Education and Research, http://www.mayoclinic.org/healthy-living/infant-and-toddler-health/expert-answers/infant-formula/faq-2005 7869, January 19, 2013.

How to Care for Your Baby's Gums and Emerging Teeth. Baby Center, http://www.baby center.com/0_how-to-care-for-your-babys-gums-and-emerging-teeth_126.bc, 2015.

How to Protect Your Baby's Teeth from Cavities. American Academy of Pediatric Dentistry, http://www. aapd.org/assets/2/7/Education_-_Caries.pdf, 2014.

Impact of Fluoride on Neurological Development in Children. Harvard T.H. Chan School of Public Health, http://www.hsph.harvard.edu/news/features/fluoride-childrens-health-grandjean-choi/, 2014.

Infant Formula and Fluorosis. Division of Oral Health, National Center for Chronic Disease Prevention and Health Promotion, http://www.cdc.gov/fluoridation/safety/infant_formula.htm, July 10, 2013.

Kids Teeth Q&A. NHS Choices, http://www.nhs.uk/Livewell/dentalhealth/Pages/Goodhabitskids.aspx, February 12, 2013.

Learn More About Floss and Interdental Cleaners. America Dental Association, http://www.ada.org/en/scie nce-research/ada-seal-of-acceptance/product-category information/ floss-and-other-interdental-cleaners, 2014.

Mottled Enamel. http://medical-dictionary.thefree dictionary.com/mottled+enamel, 2014.

Mouthrinses. Dental Health Foundation, Ireland, http://www.dentalhealth.ie/dentalhealth/teeth/mouthrinses. html, 2015.

Nanne SM. Do Easy A Four-Year-Old Can Do It! RDH, September 2014: 66, 102.

National Dental Hygiene Month, 2014. ADHA.org, http://www.adha.org/national-dental-hygiene-month, 2014.

Nelson GR. 20 Amazing Facts About Fluoride. Dimensions of Dental Hygiene, http://www.dimensionsof dentalhygiene.com/print.aspx?id=17043, July 2013.

Nelson T. The Consequences of Convenience. Dimensions of Dental Hygiene, http://www.dimensionsof dentalhygiene.com/2012/02_February/Features/The_Conse quences_of_Convenience.aspx, February 2012.

Oral Health: A Window to Your Overall Health. Mayo Clinic, http://www.mayoclinic.org/healthy-living /adult-health/in-depth/dental/art-20047475, 2015.

Oral-Systemic Health. American Dental Association, http://www.ada.org/en/member-center/oral-healthtopics/ oral-systemic-health, 2015.

Other Fluoride Products. Division of Oral Health, National Center for Chronic Disease Prevention and Health Promotion, http://www.cdc.gov/fluoridation/fluoride_prod ucts/, July 10, 2013.

Pacifiers: Are they Good for Your Baby? Mayo Foundation for Medical Education and Research, http://www.mayoclinic.org/healthy-living/infant-andtoddler -health/indepth/pacifiers/ art-20048140, September 25, 2014.

Pediatric Dental FAQ. http://www.mcgoughdent istry.com/pedo-faq.php?mode=desktop#Care_Of_Your _Childs_Teeth, 2015.

Periodontal Disease and Systemic Health. American Academy of Periodontology, http://www.perio.org/consum er/other-diseases, 2015.

Review of Fluoride: Benefits and Risks. Public Health Services, Department of Health and Human Services, http://health.gov/environment/ReviewofFluoride /MAJfind.htm, 1991.

School-Based Dental Sealant Programs. Division of Oral Health, National Center for Chronic Disease Prevention and Health Promotion, http://www.cdc.gov/ oralhealth/dental_sealant_program, July 10, 2013.

Sealants. Mouth Healthy, http://www.mouthhealthy .org/en/az-topics/s/sealants, 2014.

Seal Out Tooth Decay. National Institute of Dental and Craniofacial Research, http://www.nidcr.nih.gov/oral health/topics/toothdecay/sealouttoothdecay.htm, July 31, 2014.

Should You Rinse After Brushing Your Teeth? Oral Answers, http://www.oralanswers.com/rinse-afterbrushing/, October 3, 2011.

Slim L. Don't Ease Up! RDH, October 2014: 88-89.

Songsiripradubboon S, Hamba H, Trairatvorakul C, Tagami J. Sodium Fluoride Mouthrinse Used Twice Daily Increased Incipient Caries Lesion Remineralization in an In Situ Model. National Center for Biotechnology Information, U.S. National Library of Medicine, http://www.ncbi.nlm.nih.gov/pubmed/24394584, March 2014.

Sprague B, Bernhardt M, Barrett S. Fluoridation: Don't Let the Poisonmongers Scare You. http://www.quack watch.com/03HealthPromotion/fluoride.html, March 30, 2013.

Statement on Early Childhood Caries. America Dental Association, http://www.ada.org/ en/about-the-ada/ada-positions-policies-and-statements/statement-on-early-childhood-caries, 2014.

Sundar S. Sugar-Free Medicines are Counter-productive. National Center for Biotechnology Information, U.S. National Library of Medicine, http://www.ncbi.nl m.nih.gov/pubmed/22955756, September 2012.

Taking a Bite Out of Baby Bottle Tooth Decay. Harvard Health Publications, http://www.harvardhealth content.com/HealthCommentaries/66,COL032206, 2014.

The Tooth Decay Process: How to Reverse It and Avoid a Cavity. National Institute of Dental and Craniofacial Research, http://www.nidcr.nih.gov/oral health/OralHealthInformation/ChildrensOralHealth/Tooth DecayProcess.htm, May 2013.

Thumb Sucking: Help Your Child Break the Habit. Mayo Foundation for Medical Education and Research, http://www.mayoclinic.org/healthy-living/childrens-health/in-depth/thumb-sucking/art-20047038, September 20, 2012.

Water Fluoridation and Cancer Risk. American Cancer Society, http://www.cancer.org/cancer/cancer causes/othercarcinogens/athome/water-fluoridation-and-cancer-risk, June 24, 2013.

Yeung CA. A Systematic Review of the Efficacy and Safety of Fluoridation. National Center for Biotechnology Information, U.S. National Library of Medicine, http://www.ncbi.nlm.nih.gov/pubmed/18584000, 2008.